MW00680372

Happiness Is . . . for Nurses

Happiness Is . . . for Nurses

Humorous Situations in Nursing

Betty Gold Heil Morrison

VANTAGE PRESS
New York

Published by Vantage Press, Inc.
516 West 34th Street, New York, New York 10001

Manufactured in the United States of America
ISBN: 0-533-11689-9

Library of Congress Catalog Card No.: 95-90694

0 9 8 7 6 5 4 3 2 1

To my parents, Marie and Ray Gold, who supported me, and to my brother, Ray Gold, who encouraged me to publish this book.

To my first husband, Ronald W. H. Heil Sr., and my three sons, Ronald Jr., David, and Jeffrey, for allowing me to express my feelings and frustrations. For their support when work got me down and for laughing with me, or at me, whatever the case may be.

To my second husband, Norman Morrison, for helping me with this book. He had never had a working wife, and I wasn't going to let him get used to one. For letting me retire, about the time I was feeling "nurse burnout," so I could do other things. Now we stop and smell the roses together.

Contents

Introduction   ix

1. Nurse's Training   1
2. Working as a Registered Nurse   11
3. Emergencies   26
4. OB Patients   38
5. All in a Day's Work   51

Introduction

This book is just light reading, written mainly to make people laugh! If you have any medical background, I'm sure you will enjoy this book more. I'm not writing this book to laugh at people, but so we can laugh with people. I'm mostly laughing at myself. This is not written to hurt anyone. Everything in this book is true. All of these experiences happened while I was working as a nurse. If you are squeamish, stop now. We, who work only with sick people, have to laugh—or we will cry—and each time you cry you die a little. Laughter is our steam vent—so we can be a better nurse, doctor, or whatever.

I hope you enjoy reading this book as much as I have enjoyed writing it.

Happiness Is . . . for Nurses

1

Nurse's Training

I became a registered nurse way back when it required three years of training—with only two weeks off in the summer. We were under strict supervision and we were allowed to go home one night a month only if we had a note from Mom.

We were expected to study two hours every night and then could be out till 10:30. There were bed checks and supervision around the clock. We were not allowed in or

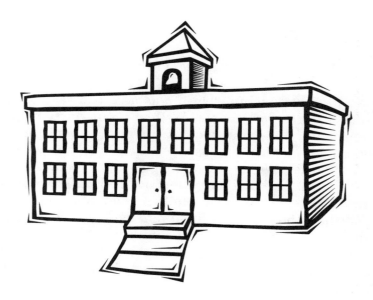

near the hospital with slacks on or our hair up in curlers. Mrs. Johnson was our watchdog. Now I know she was a very nice lady, but then we really felt very "picked on."

At 10:30 P.M. all student nurses and their boyfriends would gather on the front porch to kiss "good night"—and Mrs. Johnson would be there too. Boys were uncomfortable kissing in front of her—and she was never late, nor did she ever miss a night, nor did she go in until all her girls were safely tucked away.

We enjoyed the studies, the teachers, the hospital, the patients, and, I guess, even Mrs. Johnson.

My first day on the "floor," I timidly answered a light. The patient said, "I'd like to see a nurse." I left the room, found the supervisor, and told her the patient in 233 wanted to see a nurse.

"What are you?" she asked.

"A nurse," I answered.

"Then go answer the light."

Happiness is . . . a cheerful doctor at 3 A.M.

I worked nights when I was a second-year student with a third-year student. We had about thirty patients that night. For moral support, we always went together on rounds or when we heard a noise. One night we heard an odd noise. We ran down the hall to the room the noise came from. We found the patient on the floor. The man was about six feet three inches tall and had fallen out of bed. Somehow the two of us lifted him back into the bed and she sent me to find the night supervisor.

I tried to run quietly down the hall on rubber-soled shoes, but my starched skirt made such a noise. Later that night I got brave and went to answer a light on my own. The halls were rather dark in the middle of the night. Two patients were in that room: one asked for the bedpan and the other one was dead. I drew the curtains around the bed and gave the old man the pan.

All the time I was carrying on a silent argument with myself. *You are a nurse. Take his pulse. Maybe he just looks dead. NO WAY! He looks dead—he is dead! I will not touch him. You are a poor excuse of a nurse. Maybe so. Better run and get the supervisor. Best idea I've had all night!!!!* So with rustling skirts, I went racing for the supervisor. She came and confirmed that he was really dead. He was an old, old man and his was a very easy death.

The night was only half over. A lady who was in for a threatened miscarriage—did—and I was off and running for my helpful supervisor again.

Just at dawn, we were making rounds again. As I was shining the flashlight up to the head of the bed, my heart stopped. A patient had put on a horrible monster mask; *at that point I almost gave up nursing.* I still vividly remember that night, even after all these years.

Happiness is . . . a patient who will cheerfully follow doctor's orders.

As a student nurse, I had to work in all departments: OB, Surgery, Medical, Nursery, Kitchen, etc. While we were in Surgery, we had to be "on call."

One Sunday morning at about 4:00 A.M. I was called for a burn case. A youngish man's wife had died and he was having a hard time coping. He had drunk too much on Saturday night. While sitting in his car, he had passed out and dropped a lighted cigarette. One hand was burned rather badly.

I was just the "circulating" nurse. That meant the "scrub" nurse was sterile, and if she needed something, I

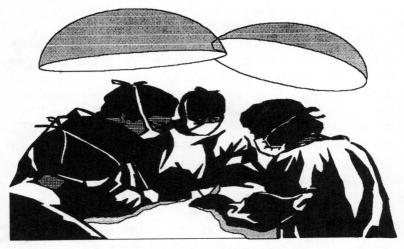

had to go and get it. The doctor took the forceps, gently lifted the top layer of skin at the wrist, and peeled it down off the fingers. Then he removed the next layer.

"Go get some air," I was told.

I went out on the "airing" porch and took deep breaths, feeling very ashamed. *Here I was a nurse, although a fairly new nurse, but still a nurse. I should not act like that!*

I marched back in, swallowing fast, and telling myself to straighten up and be a nurse! Maybe it was the smell of burnt flesh. The doctor sent me out of Surgery three times; I guess because I was looking green.

Finally the patient was wheeled out to his room. We cleaned up the Surgery, which I did fine, and went to breakfast. They were serving "fried bacon." THAT SMELL! The cook was flabbergasted when I made myself a bologna sandwich.

Happiness is ... having someone pick you up after a long hard night.

Another time in Surgery, we had an emergency appendix. As the "scrub" nurse, I was the one to hand the doctor the instruments. I had the sterile instruments all laid out on my table. I bumped the table and over went all my sterile instruments!

Oh, dear! If I could only have crawled under the table! I called on the circulating nurse to bring me a new tray of sterile instruments. Soon delivered, they had only been out of the autoclave a short time and were still warm. The rest of the surgery went without incident.

About a month later, I was called into the office. *What had I done? Or what had the office found out about me?* There was a lawyer, the head of surgery, the supervisor of nurses, and the administrator of the hospital. *All the big wheels. What had I done???* I was told to sit in a chair and answer questions, which was hard to do because of the lump in my throat and the butterflies in my stomach.

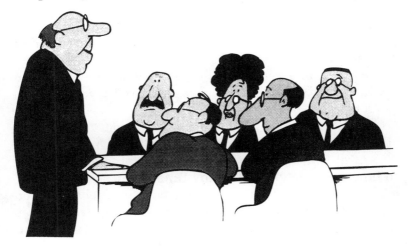

All the questions were about that surgery. *Now I was scared. Just because I was clumsy and tipped over the table, was that the cause of all this commotion?*

I finally found out what it was all about. When the doctor changed the dressings, he laughingly told the patient how the nurse had dropped the instruments on the floor and he had to operate with hot instruments. The patient went to his lawyer to sue the doctor for burns. All they wanted from me, in a roundabout way, was to know how hot the instruments were. The doctor and I would have had burnt hands if the instruments were that hot!

Happiness is . . . never being interrupted in the middle of charting.

I remember another time in Surgery, when I was the "scrub" nurse. The doctor held his hand out and the nurse slapped the instrument into his palm. Usually the surgeon does not ask for the one he wants. He expects the nurse to know. That day I was positioned near the end of the table and I could not see what they were doing. The chief surgeon would hold out his hand and I was to put what he needed into it. I didn't know what he wanted and I didn't give him what he expected.

Finally, in a very soft and deadly voice, he said, "You are not handing me what I want. Aren't you a mind reader?"

"No," I snapped back angrily, feeling very frustrated. "I'm a nurse." *Me and my big mouth. Would he report me?*

After that he asked for what he wanted and I gave it to him. I was so glad when my time in Surgery was over, and I'm sure he was too. It must be terribly hard on surgeons to break in new surgical nurses every three months. Just when you become good in one department,

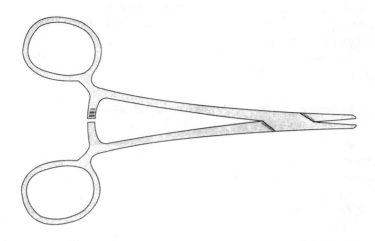

it is time to move to the next one. *I'm sure glad I ended up in OB, And I'm sure all the surgeons are too.*

Happiness is . . . a male patient who can void lying flat in bed.

Years ago we had no recovery room. We got the patient ready for surgery, took care of other patients, and then sat with our "new surgical patient" until he or she was awake after returning from surgery. We hated that, as our other patients would have to wait until the surgical patient woke up. We were always happy when a family member was there. After patients responded to their names, a family member could sit with them.

One busy morning my female patient would not wake up. I was upset, because I had other patients to care for. Finally my patient started to move around a little.

"John, John," she said.

Happily I hurried out to the hall to tell her husband

he could come in—only I had forgotten her last name. Not wanting to take time to go back and look at the chart, I said, "Uh, John, your wife is waking up. You can go in now."

His response was, "She is my wife, but my name is not John."

Happiness is . . . no admits on your shift.

As a student nurse, I was asked to do things I had never dreamed of. I answered a light one day. A male patient asked me if I would do him a big favor.

"Sure," I answered. *After all, as a nurse, I should be able to do what the patient wants.*

"Here," he said, as he spread his eyelid and dropped his glass eye out into his other hand. "Will you wash this for me?"

After I swallowed twice, I finally reached out and took his eye to wash. I'm sure he pulled similar tricks on many other young nurses with that eye.

Happiness is . . . not having to answer the same light one minute after you had just left the room.

At times, as a student nurse I was a little "gutsy." I remember, one very busy day, we had an ornery old man. I don't remember what he was in for, but he had to have one last IV and then we could take the IV out, and he was fighting us all the way. One son was standing up, holding his arm down, one hand on his wrist and one hand on his elbow. His elderly wife was patting him, brushing his hair back, wiping his face, and pleading with him to hold still. His other grown children were all hovering around him. They too were begging him to lie still just a little longer. He didn't say a word, but just lay there and as soon as the son holding his arm let up a little, he would twitch and the IV would come out.

I spent most of the afternoon checking his IV. I had to get the head nurse to restart it once, and she told me to watch it more closely. In those days, supervisors and head nurses were the only ones who could start IVs. She was as busy as we students were, and I didn't want to have to tell her the IV was out again.

Being exasperated with the whole situation, I marched in and told them all to leave and sit in the waiting room until the IV was in. The family was surprised with me! How could they leave him alone?? He'd move and the IV would come out.

I told them that he WOULD lie still and they could come back as soon as the IV was in. They left with many backward glances. The old man lay as still as a doll, the IV went in and was discontinued, and I let the family return. I was very nice to the old man because I was feeling guilty for doing what I did.

The family kept glancing at me, like "who is she who talks to Dad like that and he listens!" I'll bet he was "hell on wheels" at home. I felt very sorry for that family.

Nurses have a good sense of humor. They have to, to keep their sanity.

Happiness is . . . a patient who likes hospital food.

I remember a sweet old lady. The doctor said no bedpan; she must get up every time she had to go to the bathroom, it was too hard on her back to be on the bedpan. She also must have her shoes on, not slippers. They were black tie oxfords and very hard to get on. Like a lot of old people, she had to go often.

One night she had to go for the umpteenth time. I and another nurse went in together, and we were both struggling to get those shoes on. She felt sorry for us on our knees, struggling so hard with those hateful shoes. She looked down at us and said sweetly, *"Aren't you glad I'm not a centipede?"*

It's hard to put that kind of shoe on when you are laughing that much.

Happiness is . . . never being paged for a whole shift.

The hospital where I trained was named "Naeve Hospital" and pronounced "navy." Years ago a family with that name gave land to the hospital. We called ourselves the "Navy Beans."

Happiness is . . . time for a cup of coffee.

In the town where I took my training, we had a lot of Mexicans who came in the summer to harvest our crops. One day I was feeding a Mexican man—I don't remember what was wrong with him—and we were talking. He had a nice wife and a lot of children and he talked about them. He asked about my family and I told him I had one brother. "What did your father do—sleep?"

2

Working as a Registered Nurse

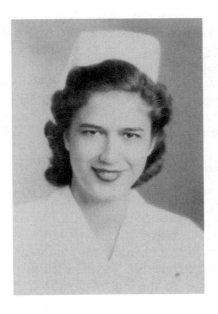

Right after finishing nurse's training, I went to the deep South to work. One day I went into a room to answer a light.

The lady had had surgery two days before. She was just closing her snuff box. She was CHEWING. I had never seen a lady chew before. I gave her what she wanted and hurried out to the head nurse, all upset.

"The lady in 807 is chewing snuff."

"I hope you gave her a container to spit in," was her calm answer.

Happiness is . . . a patient who is willing to get up and walk when he is supposed to and willing to stay in bed when he is supposed to.

Patients' care following eye surgery kept them flat in bed with their eyes bandaged for several days. I fed such a Southern gentleman from the hills of northern Georgia for many meals. He had been a rather difficult patient and let me know he didn't like "damned Yankees," of which I was one. I was pleased when he said, "I'd be proud to have you and your husband visit me and I'll even show you my still." I took that as a real compliment.

Happiness is . . . a kind word.

After working briefly in the South, I was married and moved back to Minnesota, where I stayed home for twelve years. I enjoyed being at home with my three sons until they all went to school, but I was glad to go back to nursing. I spent the next twenty years working in a small rural hospital, mostly in the Obstetrical Department.

Happiness is . . . a bashful patient, but not too bashful.

Long after graduating, I went back to visit my mother in the hospital where I was trained. She was a surgical patient there. While I was sitting with her, two student nurses came in and shyly asked me, "Are you the Betty Gold who took nurse's training here?"

"Yes," I said, very puzzled.

"We'd heard so much about you. We just had to come and see what you looked like!" they said, leaving the room.

Even as a student, I had a reputation.

Happiness is . . . extra staff when you get busy.

Later I was relearning my OB and my supervisor was named Sue. We had taken the patient into the delivery room and suddenly the baby decided to come. The doctor was on his way and I hurried to the hall to see if he was coming. He was sauntering down the hall. I didn't want to shout, so I waved my arms and gestured and did a few quick little steps, hoping he would hurry.

"Are you trying to teach me a new dance step?" he asked, not moving any faster. He delivered the baby and all ended well.

The anesthetist looked at me and shook his head. Later he said, "If he was any slower, he'd be doing yesterday's work."

Happiness is . . . if you are an OB nurse, you have long fingers.

One slow night, when I was helping out in another department, I was paged for the delivery room. I hurried down the hall and into the labor room, expecting a fat young lady to be waiting for me. There was a gray-haired, very pregnant lady, who reminded me of my aunt.

"Your first baby?" I blurted out, biting my tongue after my blunder.

"No, dear," she said in a soft voice, "my twelfth."

She had a lovely baby and the family was so thrilled, but she still looked more like a grandmother.

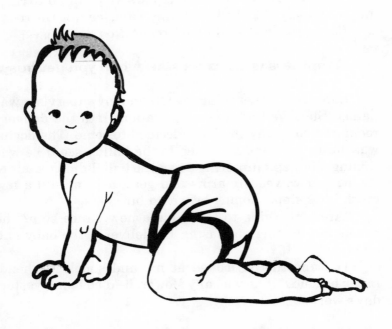

Happiness is . . . an OB who doesn't ask if she has to take her panties off.

I've been known for breaking records in the OB department. Maybe in a large hospital with residents this would not be a problem. In our little hospital, the doctor wanted to be called so he has time to come, change his clothes, scrub up and then work on the patient. Our timing sometimes was off—making the doctor unhappy and the nurse upset.

The "CHG" behind my name did mean "the

charge nurse," I really think it means "the catch hell girl."

One evening at 8:30 I had two patients in labor; both were not doing much, with mild contractions. The doctor told me not to worry as I would not have a baby on my shift. One baby was born at 10:55 P.M.; another at 11:05 P.M.; and a third OB walked in ready to deliver. Then we really had to move fast, as we only had two delivery rooms. Empty one out, clean it up, and set it up for the third baby who came at 11:32. Three babies in thirty-seven min-utes—a record that still stands today at that hospital.

I asked, "Doctor, who said I would not have any babies on my shift?"

His answer was, "A normal nurse wouldn't have."

Happiness is . . . an OB patient who doesn't push till the doctor arrives.

Several months later the day shift was having a busy time and that same doctor told the nurse to call me and see if I had driven past the hospital that morning—*I got blamed even when I wasn't there.*

Happiness is . . . never having to crawl under the bed for the patient's slippers.

Another fun night—the nursery nurses were begin-ning to object to my being in the delivery room. It seems a lot of babies were born while I was on duty, which kept them extra busy.

Four babies in three hours and eleven minutes. All that charting to do—who got what "shot" when, membranes ruptured at what time, color of fluid? So much to remember—time of birth, time and type of placenta, and kind of suture used by the doctor, etc. Lots of fun???

Well, Baby No. 1 came with the cord around its neck once—not too rare. Baby No. 2 was a footling breech, which meant the baby backed out, one leg coming out and the other leg folded up over the body. Doctors usually slid the other little leg down and then used both legs to gently pull the baby out. No one liked breech births.

Today that usually calls for a Caesarean section.

Baby No. 3 had an extremely long cord—around neck, around body, between legs and back up over body. Doctor was trying to untangle the cord from the wiggly, wet, screaming baby. He looked at me with a twinkle in his eye and said, "This kid came gift wrapped."

Baby No. 4 was a frank breech. Both legs were folded up over its body and the little bottom was coming first— another nightmare, which isn't seen much anymore. Thank goodness for C-sections. We had four healthy babies. The nursery nurse was running her legs off.

Happiness is ... not hearing the fetal heart tones for the last few minutes before birth and then hearing a loud baby's cry.

Another night I was in the delivery room. Baby was born so we were relaxed. No one else was in labor. Doctor was at work with the stitchery. A nurse called me out of the delivery room. She had rushed an OB patient up in the wheelchair and was trying to get her out of the chair and into the bed. The poor patient was holding her distended abdomen and softly moaning. I went to her side and held her till the pain went away.

"What baby is this?" I asked.

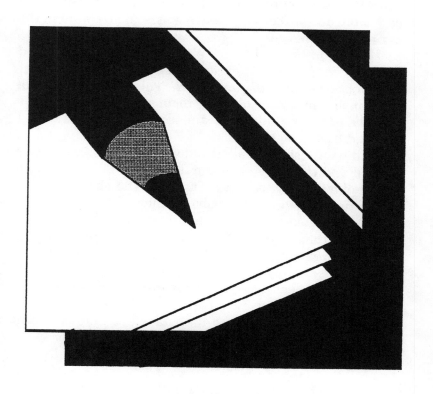

"First," she gasped.

"When did your labor start?"

"This is my third pain—with the first one, my husband called the doctor. The second one was while we were in the car and now this one."

I thought to myself—*WOW, first few contractions and carrying on like this. What will she be like in hard labor? This looks like a real fun night!!* This was the kind of patient that made the delivery room such a challenge. We quickly got her undressed and settled into bed and I checked her.

"Mary," I said, "Call the doctor—she is completely dilated and the baby is on the doorstep." This doctor, no friend of mine, argued with Mary over the phone.

"I just talked to her husband a few minutes ago," he said, "and he said her labor had just started. The nurse must be wrong. She can't be ready yet. No one goes that fast!" I guess we sounded desperate because he finally came.

"All right, I'm here—where is the patient you nurses think is about to deliver?" he asked gruffly as he burst into the labor room. Mary, who had stayed to help and was treating the newborn's eyes, said sweetly, "Doctor, your patient is across the hall and this is her baby. We delivered her!"

It is a nice feeling, at times, to know you are right.

Happiness is . . . fresh coffee when you have a minute to drink it.

One evening, as I came up from an uninterrupted dinner, I noticed the Emergency Room wheelchair outside the labor room door. It wasn't there when I went down to eat, so being nosy, I went back into the labor room.

There, in bed, was a lady definitely in hard labor. *You recognize the sights and sounds quickly when you have worked there as long as I had.* I heard noises in the delivery room.

"Mary," I called.

"I'm hurrying. I'm setting up the delivery room as fast as I can," she replied.

"Mary, come now," I called calmly, though I was far from calm! Many thoughts went through my head. *Who is this lady and who is her doctor? Who brought her to the labor room and where are the sterile gloves?* That was a silly thought. I delivered a nice healthy baby, of course, without gloves, but also without sterile drapes and not in the delivery room.

Seems like the doctor from a small town about twenty miles away had checked her at his office and decided she was in advanced labor. He brought her in his own car. He met Mary in the hall as he raced her toward the delivery room in the wheelchair. He told Mary to set up the delivery room and he went to change his clothes.

Because I was nosy and checked out that wheelchair, I delivered the baby.

Happiness is . . . a full half hour to eat without interruptions.

I really enjoyed the delivery room, but I did not like to deliver babies. Sometimes it was hard to get the mother, the doctor, the anesthetist, the father, and me all in the same room under sterile conditions at the moment the baby decided to come. And, after you had the whole crowd there, sometimes the mother's labor would stop.

Why? Who knows? So we would all stand around and wait. Some doctors did not like that and all nurses got very nervous, but then suddenly it would be all over. A very red-faced screaming baby arrived and all of us had silly grins on our faces.

Happiness is . . . never getting a note about charting from the record room.

We had Mexicans coming up from Mexico every spring to harvest the asparagus crop. Most didn't speak English and I didn't speak their language, but there were times when I wished I could say, "NO PUSHA." One day I delivered a Mexican lady. This baby was her nineteenth pregnancy. I called the doctor, knowing he would not make it on time.

When the doctor did arrive, he asked me, "Did you *really* expect me to get here on time?"

Happiness is ... going home and then not having to worry if you charted this or that.

One night I admitted an OB. She was a very scared young girl. She sat crosslegged on the bed, looking like a very pregnant Buddha. To calm her down, I was filling out our two pages of questions. Some of the questions were, "Name, address, telephone, husband's name, place of business," etc, etc.

This poor little mother-to-be was still uptight.

Next question, "Religion?"

"No," she answered and looked very puzzled.

"No religion?" I said, trying not to look surprised.

She giggled and said, "I thought you said 'virgin'!" She must have thought she really had a dumb nurse.

We got along fine after that and several hours later, she delivered a lovely baby boy.

Happiness is ... an accurate narcotic count.

I have, at times, worked in other departments. One night I was in ICU (intensive care unit). There, I was just a "gofor;" "go for this" and "go for that": answer lights, give bedpans, do blood pressures, etc.

I was giving a "heart" patient a backrub. As I was working, he was talking. "Haven't seen you around before. Are you new? You sure give a super backrub."

"Yes, I'm new here," I answered. *New to ICU, twenty years in the hospital.*

21

The poor ICU nurse was listening to our conversation and she finally joined into our conversation, saying, laughingly, <u>"She isn't new here—she came over on the Mayflower."</u>

Happiness is . . . never having to chart.

Naming babies has always fascinated me. I worked one Fourth of July and tried to help the laboring mothers name their new little ones. This helped take their minds off their labor pains.

"Sammy"—named after Uncle Sam or "Betsy" named after
    Betsy Ross. No one listened to me.
"Columbus" or "Maria" for Santa Maria for Columbus Day.
"Valentino" for Valentine's Day.
"Noel," "Holly," "Nicole," and others for Christmas.
"Eve" or "Eva" for New Year's Eve.
"Robert" or "Roberta" for Robert E. Lee.
"Abe" or "Linc" for Abraham Lincoln.
"George" or "Georgette" for George Washington.
"Autumn" for Fall.
"April" for Spring.
"Joe" for G. I. Joe for Veterans Day.
"Martin" or "Martina" for Martin Luther King Day.
"Patrick" or "Patricia" for St. Patrick's Day. And many
    more.

We had an anesthetist named John who always tried to talk the moms into naming their baby boys after him. One day I asked him, "John, who in their right mind would name a baby after a toilet?"

Had one mom name her baby Abner—would have been Daisy if baby was a girl. Al Capp, are you listening?

22

Happiness is ... a patient who will open his mouth willingly when being fed.

Late one afternoon an OB came in. *My unfavorite doctor again.* This lady was expecting her seventh child but not for two more weeks, but she was already in mild labor. I called the doctor to see if I could admit her.

"No—she isn't due for two weeks; she isn't in labor."

"Can I keep her here for an hour to watch her?" I asked.

"If it will make you feel better—go ahead, but don't get her ready for delivery."

After an hour—the contractions were still mild. *No change—but I had that "feeling."*

I called him back and asked if I could prep her for delivery.

"Since there is no change, send her home."

"Can I keep her another hour just to watch her?"

"You are so antsy when someone is in labor. Keep her if it will make you feel better."

After another hour, contractions were still mild, but somehow or other, I talked him into letting me prep her for the delivery. About an hour later, I called the doctor to come and deliver the baby of this mother who was not due for two weeks and was not even in labor.

He came and delivered the baby and never said a word about my "feeling" or about my being antsy.

The rest of the night I had to listen to the father brag about how wonderful this doctor was—how smart a man he was—how great he was. *Little did he know or could I tell him how he almost had to deliver his own son. Nor could I tell him of my arguments I had with that wonderful, marvelous, and thoughtful doctor.*

Happiness is . . . a nurse with warm hands.

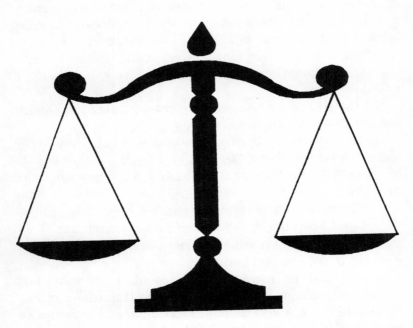

We always weighed the nursing babies before they went to breast and afterwards to see how much milk they got from Mom. I don't believe they do that anymore.

One night I was relieving in the nursery when a new father came to the door. "May I ask you a question?" he asked shyly.

"Sure."

"How do you weigh them?"

"Just put them on the scale"—thinking that was a rather dumb question.

"What kind of a scale?"

"Just a regular scale"—more dumb questions.

"Don't they fall off?"

"No, you kind of hold them on."

He looked very puzzled and then suddenly the light dawned, "Oh, you weigh the babies—I thought you weighed the breasts."

We both had a good laugh.

Happiness is . . . only giving intramuscular shots to heavy people.

Happiness is . . . only having to "stick" a patient one time for an IV.

Happiness is . . . being discharged a day sooner than you expected.

3

Emergencies

One day on the medical/surgical floor we admitted a patient about 3:00 P.M. He had been at the country club and was knocked out when hit in the head by a golf ball. He was awake and alert when brought in by the ambulance. We served our evening meal around 5:15 P.M. I carried his tray in to him.

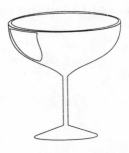

"Dinner—now!" he exclaimed. "This is much too early. I'd like a couple cocktails now and then you can bring the tray in at about seven."

Some people do not understand the hospital is not the country club or a fancy restaurant. I tried calmly to explain that the kitchen closed at 7:00 P.M. And that the doctor had not ordered cocktails for him. Everyone eats at the same time.

"I couldn't eat now. I'm not used to eating this early.

I'll not eat tonight—TAKE THE TRAY AWAY!" he replied, very angrily!

I did take his tray away, and I sure hope he was really hungry by breakfast time. I do not like to be talked to like that or in that tone of voice. I did not make the rules. Hope he did not give the night nurses too bad a time.

Some day I'm going to have surgery—a pedal-oralectomy (removal of my foot from my mouth). *I have been known to blurt out things before I think—do you do that?*

Happiness is . . . an empty tray table when you bring in the dinner tray.

Happiness is . . . a warm bedpan.

Happiness is . . . the first voiding after surgery.

Happiness is . . . a "dock" day that is also a holiday.

My friendly doctor has a tendency to be a little lazy—don't we all?

We had a threatened abortion come in. That doesn't mean she did something to try to lose the baby. It only means that for some unknown reason she was in danger of losing her baby.

This was her fifth pregnancy and she was two months along. The doctor put her on bed rest and she was fine. After several days he let her up to go to the bathroom. She started to bleed and so she was put back to bed rest. She told me she couldn't stay in bed for the next seven months, not with four little ones at home. She wished she could get up and if she lost the baby, she would feel bad, but those babies at home needed her more.

I told the doctor her wishes when he made rounds.

"Oh, you women—always having problems—always complaining. Some want to stay in bed—some don't. You women, we never can please you!"

I saw red and opened my big mouth. "If you men would lay off us women, we wouldn't have very many problems!!!"

He laughed at me—went to visit his patient and gave her bathroom privileges. She lost that baby but was back a year later to deliver a nice big healthy boy.

Happiness is . . . a rainy day when you have to work and sunshine on your day off.

I rode the ambulance many, many times to the Mayo Clinic in Rochester, Minnesota. The only time the ambulance driver asked me how fast I wanted to go was when I had a laboring mom who was only about seven months along. OBs seem to make them very nervous!

I was asked to lecture to the ambulance drivers on what to do if a baby came when they were transporting a "soon-to-be mom." I really enjoyed that and they even paid me for lecturing. *Most people do not pay me for talking.*

Happiness is . . . visitors who leave on time.

One time we raced the stork to Rochester and won by twenty minutes—really no race at all. I had been teasing the driver for several months to let me drive. I took the same EMT class the men did, but I never got to drive the ambulance. I really was only teasing.

After we left the patient with the emergency room nurses, I went to wash my hands. When I came out, the driver was in the passenger seat and he motioned me to get in the driver's seat.

Wow! I had never driven a Cadillac before. We started out and that baby really handled nice.

"How fast can I go?" I asked him.

"Fast as you want—only you pay your own fine if the police pick us up."

"I'm going to floor it just once and then I'll keep within the speed limit," I replied. "If I get picked up—you quickly get in the back and look sick."

He said, "How sick?"

"Oh, I don't know, cut your wrist or something," I answered.

I stayed within the speed limit the rest of the way home. At that time, our hospital was not used to female ambulance drivers and I drove up right at noon. Nurses and doctors eating their lunch rushed out when they saw me drive in. They thought the driver was sick.

Happiness is . . . a fractured hip that doesn't weigh three hundred pounds.

My doctor friend came out of a patient's room one night in a frenzy. His face was red and he was steaming.

"Now what?" I asked.

"Would you believe—that father in there—I don't believe it—I really don't believe it!"

Seems a young girl had a baby, and because of complications, a C-section was done. She was not married, so her daddy—the new grandpa—had to pay the bill. We did not know it then, but this was the second baby "granddad" had to pay for. Another unmarried daughter also had a baby. Grandpa was rather angry about all these doctor bills, especially with the extra cost of surgery this time.

When the doctor made rounds that evening,

"Grandpa" asked him to change the diagnosis—to make it "Removal of a tumor."

The doctor said, "A tumor with legs."

Happiness is . . . an enema that doesn't turn into a rectal douche.

One Sunday I was sent off the OB floor to work on the Medical floor. We had an old man who was very congested. The doctor's orders were to give a certain medicine and to turn the patient on his stomach; then with cupped hands, gently pound on his back to break loose the congestion, so he could cough it up.

The halls were full of visitors. The orderly and I were pounding away, trying to break loose the phlegm.

"Please don't hit me again," begged the old man with a quaking voice.

When we walked out into the hall, we were really given some nasty looks.

Happiness is . . . patients who brush their own teeth.

Another busy afternoon. Weather was very hot. A patient suddenly turned "sour" on the floor and we rushed her to ICU. I stayed in ICU lending them an extra pair of hands for the special care this patient needed. She finally stabilized, so I returned to the floor.

I answered an old, senile, confused and extremely upset lady's light. As I was trying to calm her down, she suddenly became very hostile. She had a Foley catheter in and a nearly full Foley bag. She grabbed the catheter and swung and the bag struck me on my chest—*and it broke.* An instant yellow smelly shower—on a hot summer's day.

I don't know how much urine a uniform can absorb, but it was enough. The rest dripped down into my shoes.

I got another nurse to come and try to calm her down. I headed for the linen room to get a "scrub gown" and planned to take a shower. Except a "Doctor 99" was paged three doors down from where I was. As I'm an instructor of CPR, "smelly" me responded.

"Dr. 99" means it is an emergency and all nurses who are fairly free must go directly to where the help is needed. I got up on the bed and began CPR. Someone opened all the windows. We worked on the patient for almost an hour, but it was hopeless. We weren't surprised—he had many things wrong with him.

By the time I left the room, I was drenched with sweat. My "Right Guard" had left much earlier. After CPR and the "let down" feeling you get when you lose a patient, I felt too tired to move. My arms felt like lead.

As I walked down the hall, heading for the shower, an OB walked in and from the sounds she was making, I knew I would be needed. She was a "graveda 5"—which meant her fifth pregnancy. I set up the delivery room while another nurse took care of the patient. She delivered within minutes after being admitted to the floor.

The baby was the only one who did not complain about my smell. By this time my uniform was becoming a little stiff.

It is hard to understand a doctor who is giving orders for the new mother with his hand over his mouth and holding his nose. I should have won the "award of the month" for being the "smelliest" nurse.

The next morning the old senile lady was transferred to the lock-up room for her own safety. Because she was combative, we got two male workers to escort her. When they came out of the elevator, she started to scream, "Rape! Rape! Rape!"

She really got them upset. *Never a dull moment!!!*

Happiness is . . . someone to talk to after a patient dies.

I have always worked the 3:00 P.M. to 11:30 P.M. shift. We called ourselves, *"The ladies of the night."*

Happiness is . . . a full supply cupboard.

When the hospital heard I was going to write a book, my friendly doctor asked me if he would recognize himself in it. Since he and I have had a few rounds together, I said, "You'd better believe you will!!!"

Happiness is . . . the patient who was given two ounces of castor oil also has bathroom privileges.

As student nurses, we learned all about the "Sippy Diet" invented by Dr. Sippy for ulcer patients. We used to wonder if he was married and had a wife named Mrs. Sippy?

Happiness is . . . enough Geri chairs for all the Geriatric patients.

Happiness is . . . a correct "I and O" slip at the end of a shift.

I'm an instructor for CPR and a dear friend asked me to go with her to her Catholic Church. I was to give a quick class in CPR to the ushers. Since the church was right next

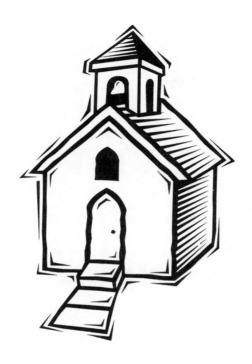

door to the hospital, they figured that the ushers should
know a little bit about CPR to help the patient until they
could get a doctor.

Mary and I held a class for about fifteen ushers. The
next day that priest asked Mary if I was Catholic.

"No, she's Lutheran."

"Why did she offer to teach the class?"

"Father, nurses do not care what a person's religion
is."

"Since she did that, I think we should buy her a box
of candy."

Mary, who is rather heavy, thinks everyone else is too.

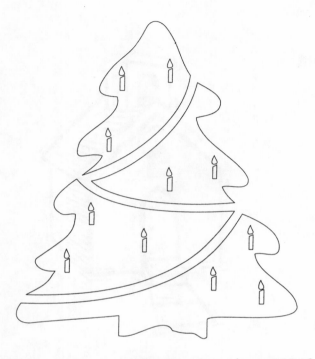

She suggested a five-dollar gift certificate would be better.
A few days later, I met that priest at the hospital.

"Thank you, Father, for the nightgown you gave me
for services rendered."

Happiness is . . . an IV that stays on time.

**Happiness is . . . an OB that doesn't scream from
3 cm on.**

**Happiness is . . . a patient who doesn't mind be-
ing awakened for pills, temperatures, or blood pressures, etc. (whatever the doctor ordered).**

I'm not a Catholic, but I got to know several "Fathers." One priest was a small, wiry, elderly man who would come to the hospital every day to bless our new mothers. He came one Christmas Eve while I was on duty.

"God bless all you mothers who work Christmas Eve," he said.

"Father, how about blessing all the daddies who have to stay home with all their excited children waiting for Mom and Santa Claus?"

"God bless you, my child, for thinking of them. I'm going to bless your most used muscle."

"Father, on me it is my tongue."

He laughed and blessed my tongue that Christmas Eve. How many of you have a blessed tongue?

Happiness is . . . finding a "full" chux and a dry sheet.

My three sons had heard me talk "hospital" talk with my husband.

The youngest one was about five when he started his science lesson at the dinner table. "Mom, babies come from eggs." A fact he picked up someplace. The two older boys started to giggle.

"They get into your tummy and you grow big and fat. You go to the hospital and the doctor helps get the baby out." Another fact.

Then he looked very puzzled. "Mommie, what do you nurses do with all those egg shells?"

My dear husband looked at me and, in a very serious voice, said, "Mommie, you work there, you tell him."

Happiness is . . . the brown spot on your uniform is chocolate.

When a patient arrived a few minutes before the change of shift and you admitted him, you had to finish the job before you went off duty. That could mean overtime. Overtime for a student just meant you worked till your work was done.

One night a "bum" was admitted. Now they are called "street people." "Sailor Sam," as he was called, was turned over to me to be admitted. I do not know how he got that nickname. He looked like a pudgy little man. I was to help him undress and get into a hospital gown.

This was in the fall of the year in Minnesota. First, I peeled off a pair of coveralls and a flannel shirt, then another pair of bib overalls and another shirt. A pair of jeans and another shirt came off next. The next layers were (1) a pair of two-piece long underwear, (2) a pair of one-piece long underwear, (3) a pair of jockey shorts and a t-shirt, each set a size smaller.

Now I had a little bird of a man who definitely needed a bath. Needless to say, I did not get off on time.

Happiness is . . . a patient who does not need four baths before you put him into bed.

As the years went by, some patients did not get cleaner. A Candy Striper (volunteer) took a tray into ICU. She came out looking very puzzled. "Why do nurses bathe a patient with his stockings on?"

"I'll check," I said. I went into ICU and the nurses were scrubbing the patient's feet. He did not have stockings on—only very, very dirty feet.

"You'll have to forgive me for being so dirty. I don't

have a wife," he told the nurses!!!! *Is it really a wife's job to bathe her husband?*

Happiness is . . . a patient with clean toenails.

4

OB Patients

One morning, when they had three mothers in labor, I was called to come in as an extra—only until a few babies were born. As I walked into the labor room where the doctor and the OB supervisor were, the doctor said, "Good, you are here—now maybe we will get some action!"

Everyone knew when I'm on duty—things happen. The supervisor gave me a dirty look as she thought the doctor was unhappy with her work, but he was just teasing me. Two hours later I went home, three babies had been born, the doctor was in his office, and I hope the supervisor was happy.

Happiness is . . . a noisy, confused patient who sleeps through the whole night.

Some doctors have a very dry sense of humor. A new young mother—about nineteen years old—had very bad hemorrhoids. They were so swollen and so terribly painful. When her doctor came, I told him about her. I gave him a rubber glove and lubricant. We went into her room together and he very carefully put the hemorrhoids back in.

"Now, hang her up by her heels till tomorrow," he said in a very serious voice.

"But, Doctor, it is so hard to swallow in that position. May I take her down for meals?" I asked.

"Yes," he said as he walked out.

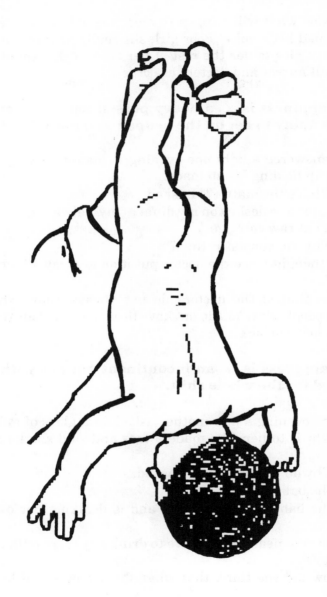

"Now what will happen to me?" she asked in a very frightened little voice. Poor girl, she really believed us. I was very nice to her the rest of her stay so she wouldn't think all nurses and doctors are crazy.

Happiness is . . . a heavy person who can raise up his fanny to get on the bedpan and not miss it.

I answered a light one evening. A man was lying all curled up holding his stomach.

"What's the matter?" I asked.

"I ate the coleslaw on my dinner tray. I always get sick when I eat raw cabbage."

"Why did you eat it then?"

"I thought since the doctor put it on my tray, I had to eat it."

I explained the doctors do not always know what makes people sick. You do not have to eat food on your tray if it makes you sick.

Happiness is . . . an incontinent patient with a dry bed for the whole shift.

One evening a new mother asked for a glass of milk. I brought it to her. She made a face and said she hated milk.

"Why do you drink it?" I asked.

"The baby needs it."

"The baby is two days old and is drinking her own milk."

"Do you mean I don't have to drink any more milk for the baby?"

How did she think that what she drank would help

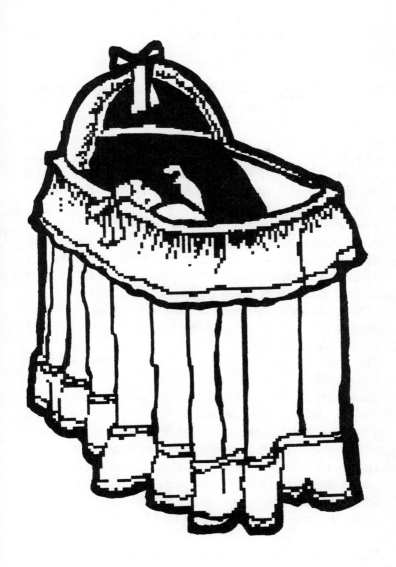

her baby when she wasn't nursing? She was trying to be a good mother.

Happiness is ... an order to discontinue an IV—just after you have found it infiltrated.

Sometimes doctors can be so unreasonable—when you call them at 11:00 P.M. for an order, they are angry because you did not ask them at 8:00 P.M. when they made rounds. We would have, if the patient had made his request known then.

A very short-fused doctor made rounds at tray time. He really chewed all the nurses out. He went to see one of his patients who was not supposed to get out of bed. When he found her sitting up in a chair, he came out to the nurse's station and really screamed at us. *We did not watch his patients. We just stood around and talked. We were unreliable, incompetent, and undependable, etc., etc., etc.* His red face set off his white hair.

After he left I went to the patient's room and just chatted with her.

"Did a nurse help you up into the chair?" I asked.

"Oh no, dear," she answered. "I was so tired of the bed I just decided to sit in the chair for a while."

I helped her back to bed and tried to explain to her that the doctor wanted her to stay in bed. The doctor could have done the same thing.

Sometimes I think the doctors believe we stay awake nights thinking of things to make them angry.

Happiness is ... a handy emesis basin.

Happiness is ... when off duty, not having to

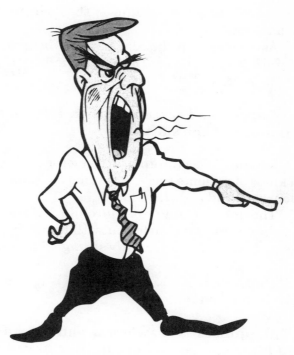

**listen to people describing their operations, ill-
nesses, or labors or those of any of their families.**

One night we were short of nurses and long on patients. A delivered OB put her light on. She was going home
the next day, as she had delivered three days earlier. She
was on welfare. *Sometimes welfare patients demand the
most attention and will be the first to complain about you.*

We had had a couple of emergencies and several very
sick patients plus all the other patients on the floor. I was
scared as I hurried down the hall. Something must be
wrong for her to call for help.

"I dropped my magazine on the floor. Would you pick it up for me?"

As I picked up the magazine, I thought, *This is the time to bite your tongue. Thank goodness, most patients are not like that.*

Happiness is . . . an IV with 1000 cc in it at the beginning of the shift.

One day I was working on the second floor. There were all kinds of patients there, including children. I had to give a four-year-old a shot.

The mother said to the child, "Here comes that naughty nurse who hurts you with those shots." *Needless to say, I could have cheerfully strangled that mother.*

Happiness is . . . a child who hugs you after you give him a "shot."

Happiness is . . . when a patient wants a hypo and after you go and get it, they have turned over and are ready for it.

We had a clinic in our town with about twelve doctors. In the evenings they took turns making rounds. If an OB came in and her doctor was not on call, she had to take the one who was. Sometimes the doctor would write on the chart, "When this patient comes in, call me and not the doctor on call." *That was fine but usually the doctor's wife answered—and gave you a hard time. "He is not on call tonight. Why do you bother him on his evening off, etc."*

You have to very calmly and politely explain to her that he wants to be called. His orders are to call him. Would she please give him the message and see what he says?

Sometimes you get the feeling that doctors and wives think you are put on earth just to make their lives miserable!

One night a good friend and fellow nurse came in about 7:00 P.M. in labor. This was her fourth child, and she had always had very short and easy deliveries. She said her doctor had promised to deliver her. I called him. He wasn't on call and his wife answered.

"No, you can't talk to him. We are leaving tomorrow at 5:00 A.M."

"But I'm sure she will deliver before 9:00 P.M. and he did promise her!" The wife would not let me talk to him and since she repeated everything I said, I felt sure the doctor was right there with her.

I had to tell my friend her doctor could not deliver her as I could not reach him. *Small white lie?* I calmed her down, as she was crying. I convinced her that the doctor on call was just as good. *In fact, the doctor on call who did deliver her was better, in my opinion.* She was an ICU nurse, so she did not know a lot about OB doctors.

All nurses should go to Heaven because they have caught enough Hell on earth.

Happiness is . . . an IV stays in as long as it is supposed to.

One Saturday morning I went to the hospital book sale at 8:00 A.M. I saw a minister hurrying across the parking lot. *I wondered if a patient was dying.*

After I had bought my books, I went into the dining room to have coffee with the nurses on their break.

"Someone dying? I saw a minister hurrying across the parking lot when I came."

"No," the third-floor nurse said laughingly. "We really had a fun and different morning."

45

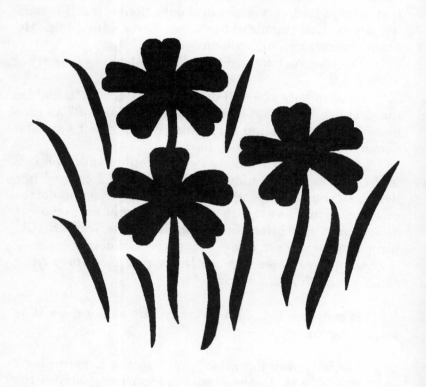

This couple had planned a big church wedding. They had sent out invitations, had the minister and the church ready for that Saturday afternoon. But the bride went into labor early that morning. They decided to get married before the baby was born. The groom, and new father-to-be, made several phone calls. The best man and the maid of honor got there in the nick of time.

The ward secretary ran around to all the rooms, and if patients had flowers, she asked for one from each. She made a bouquet. The minister married them while the patient was in bed in hard labor. The wedding was stopped once and all were sent out of the room so the OB nurse could check her. But the Lutheran minister didn't shorten the wedding ceremony. Twenty minutes after they became man and wife, she delivered a lovely baby girl. That girl almost was a flower girl at her parents' wedding. Never a dull moment on the third floor.

Happiness is . . . a patient admitted two hours before your shift ends, not two minutes.

Happiness is . . . a patient who can hold his leg stiff when you put on his elastic stockings.

Happiness is . . . a good ward secretary.

Twins weren't born very often in our little hospital. One night, I admitted an OB who had been told by her doctor that she would have twins.

Her whole family was so excited. Grandpa had gone out and bought twin cribs, high chairs, etc.

When she delivered, she had only one big healthy baby boy. *What a let down!*

Another time, the night nurses arrived just in time

to take over the delivery room as I was going off duty. I had admitted this lady, who was expecting one baby.

Before going home, I went back to the delivery room to see what she had. The doctor was saying, "A nice healthy little boy."

The mom said, "Oh, I kind of wanted a girl."

"Hang on," said the doctor. "You have a chance of getting a girl. There is another one in here."

She did have another one. But it was a boy. Both parents were surprised and happy. The doctor had not predicted twins, and we were all very surprised and happy for them.

That's the closest I ever came to helping deliver twins!

Happiness is . . . a posy jacket that does.

Happiness is . . . a patient who can hold an enema.

One night, the emergency room nurse called up to the third floor. They needed our help. A young lady, very pregnant, walked in. The first question is always, "Who is your doctor?"

"I don't have one," was the answer. *Wow, no prenatal care.*

"Do you know you are pregnant?" the nurse asked, feeling foolish to ask such a question.

"Yes," was the answer. "I was hoping it would go away if I ignored it." *When this happened years ago, unwed mothers weren't accepted as readily as they are now.*

Then she said, "I'll tell you how I got pregnant."

We looked at each other; *did we really want to hear this?*

"I was riding in the front seat of the car, with my

48

boyfriend driving," she continued. "It was a very dark night. There was no moon and my boyfriend hit a dog and I became pregnant."

We couldn't argue with her; we weren't there. After that, whenever my husband and I were driving on a dark night, I would caution him about hitting a dog.

Would hitting a cat produce the same results?

Happiness is . . . never having to use your liability insurance.

For a bladder infection, the doctor wanted a midstream sample of urine. The patient asked, "You want me to catch it on the run?"

Happiness is . . . patients who let you know their wants early in the evening so their doctor can be notified.

One slow evening after we got the patients settled for the night and were doing our charting, a job all nurses hate, the elevator door opened. An older man and young man got out pushing a wheelchair. They were both really dressed up, and the young lady in the wheelchair had on a wedding dress. This floor was the OB floor, and we usually don't get ladies in wedding dresses.

She was holding her nose, crying and screaming, "I can't breathe, I can't breathe!!!"

After her wedding, while she was surrounded by guests, she had bent down to check her shoe. At that moment, a small niece jumped up and hit her right on the nose. Such a painful thing to happen on your wedding night.

"Please help me, I can't breathe."

49

We told her to breathe through her mouth, as she had been doing all the time. She calmed down but was still in pain. We sent them back to the emergency room on the first floor. I don't know how they got past the emergency room or why they pushed the third floor button.

We all had a good laugh because as they wheeled her back into the elevator, they were arguing over who should pay the emergency room bill.

The young man thought Daddy should, and the daddy said, "No way, she's yours now!"

Happiness is . . . a nasal oxygen cannula that stays in the nose, not under the chin.

5

All in a Day's Work

One doctor in our town was noted for his poor handwriting. One evening, while making rounds, he wrote three orders on a patient's chart. He left and the ward secretary started to transfer the orders—only she couldn't read the last order. We tried and tried—all the nurses on the floor. Finally we gave up and I called the doctor. I told him the patient's name and read him the first two orders—and asked him about the third one. Only three words—but what did they say?

He couldn't remember what he had ordered, so he told us to chart "Cancel third order." He would try to figure it out in the morning on A.M. rounds. The patient wasn't too ill, so this didn't jeopardize her recovery. After that, whenever he wrote any orders, he would ask if there was a nurse here who could read handwriting.

I said sure, if I knew a doctor who could write. As the years went by, more and more doctors wrote poorly, so we accused that doctor of giving bad penmanship lessons.

Happiness is . . . doctor's orders you can read.

I was helping out on the third floor and went around taking temperatures and blood pressures. I went into a room where there was a middle-aged male patient and a male visitor. After I was done with my work, he said, "Wait, I really have a good story to tell you."

"Is it dirty?" I asked. By the way he was smiling, I knew it was.

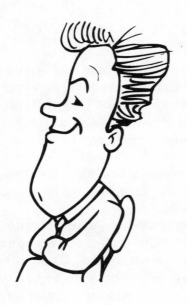

"Boy, is it ever," was his gleeful answer.

"Good, tell me as soon as I close the door," I said. I went to the door—walked out and closed the door behind me. *I resent men who think they can say anything they want to nurses and we are supposed to like it.*

Happiness is . . . a patient who can wait on himself.

We had a very good OB nurse. She could take care of a patient and be able to tell when the baby would be born.

I never tried to guess and tell the patient when her baby would come. If I was off an hour, it was just too hard on the patient. The patient would think she could hold out that long and if the time went over, the pains would seem to be more than she could bear. But this nurse could do it with perfect results. She came in to have her fourth child.

She told me the time the baby would be born—and was three minutes off. *The OB doctors love a nurse like that.*

Happiness is . . . a patient with a normal temperature.

We had a young male nurse at our hospital for a few months. In those days there were not many male nurses and none at our hospital until he came. He had been discharged from the army and later went to a large city hospital. One day he was on "meds." That meant he gave all the medications on that floor.

The young male nurse had to give a senile little old lady patient a "pain shot." She and her two elderly sisters lived together. She was the eldest and the sisters were pretending they were taking care of her at home. She did not know she wasn't at home. They didn't want us to use the word "shot." The nurse brought the hypo into the room. One of the sisters said, "Turn over, dear, here comes the nice young man with the little prick."

The young male nurse thought the old lady was talking dirty.

Happiness is . . . no emergencies.

We were told to describe all things affecting the patients. This resulted in some funny charting by new student nurses:

"Patient complaining of having a hot head and cold feet."
"Barn red blood."
"Chunky pea green emesis."

Happiness is . . . instant urine when you catheterize a patient.

After being a mother and housewife for twelve years, I went back to work. Boy, did I have a lot to learn. We had boiled everything—needles, syringes, tubes, etc. I was an

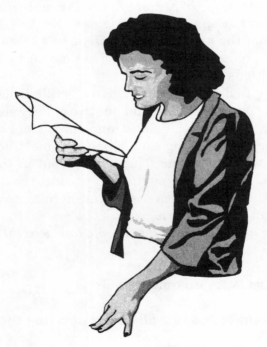

expert on boiling, but now they didn't even need that skill anymore. Now everything was disposable, so much had changed.

One evening I came out of a patient's room and said to the nurses who were charting, "That wife is in bed with her husband." *Thinking, boy we never used to allow that.*

"Which patient?" asked a doctor who was sitting nearby. He seemed very upset, so I quickly thought of the diagnosis—nothing contagious. So I said, again without thinking, "It's okay, he is in traction."

Boy, did everyone laugh at me.

Happiness is . . . an IV that goes in the first time.

I was called to ride ambulance one night about 2:00 A.M. A nineteen-year-old man was on a motorcycle and a van had hit him from the side so that his leg was crushed between the car bumper and his cycle.

The doctor in our emergency room put a tourniquet on his leg and sent us racing to the Mayo Clinic in Rochester, Minnesota, only thirty-odd miles away.

About ten miles out, the young man came to a little. He knew his leg was really hurting, so he tried to get up. I had my hands full, trying to keep him on the cot, watching the IV and his leg. No free hands to help you keep your balance as you raced through the night. My orders were to loosen the tourniquet twice on the way.

When we got to the emergency room at Mayo, several doctors were waiting for us. "Who put this tourniquet on this leg? Don't you know it can damage the foot?" one shouted at me.

"Our doctor did," I answered.

"Remove it," he yelled. No one made a move, so I stepped forward and took it off. Blood spurted out from all the severed arteries and veins in the leg, making many little fountains.

"Put it on—put it back on!" he yelled.

That young man would have bled to death long before we could have gotten him to the hospital without the tourniquet.

"Prepare him for surgery. Add another bottle to the IV. Put in a Foley catheter," he shouted. All the doctors were jumping to do his orders. I wondered if he was hard of hearing or if all the other doctors who worked there were deaf.

The young man had been out drinking beer and his bladder was very full. The "Foley" was disconnected, so when it was inserted, the pressure in the full bladder sprayed urine all over the doctors.

My ambulance team and I were on our way out the door when the last thing we heard was the doctor scream- ing to stop the urine. We laughed all the way home. *I was so glad that doctor did not work at our hospital.*

The young man had to have his leg taken off. No one was surprised. The last I heard he was playing softball with his new leg and doing very well.

Happiness is .... a doctor who orders all the things a patient might need every time he admits a patient.

When I went to work the next afternoon, I was very stiff and sore. Trying to keep your balance in a racing ambulance when your hands are busy with the patient makes you use your legs. You even try to dig your toes into the floor. That's hard to do with shoes on.

"Boy, am I stiff and sore today," I said. One of the nurses who heard me wanted to know why.

"From working last night," I answered.

"I worked last night and I'm not stiff and sore." Since I was a widow then, she always tried to read something into everything I did after my husband was killed. "What were you doing after work last night?" she asked with a smirk.

"It wasn't the two older men that bothered me. It was that nineteen-year-old that I couldn't keep up with," I told her as I walked away.

Boy, was she busy all evening trying to find out about the nineteen-year-old I was out with. She wouldn't ask me and finally the other nurses told her.

A month later I sent myself a rose at the hospital on a day I knew she would be working. She saw the rose in the vase and the card addressed to me. She opened the card and read it. All I had written on the card was. "Thanks for last night, John." I told no one about the rose, so no one knew what it meant. She sure was busy all evening trying to find out. She never asked me.

I do not like people trying to find out all about my social life. For five years I had no social life. Then I met a man and started to date. However, I will say about that nurse, if I had ever gotten sick, I would like her to care for me. She was a very good nurse!

Happiness is . . . when a patient drops a glass, it is empty and made of paper.

One night, my new friend and I were at a very nice restaurant. A couple of tables away, I saw a couple I thought I knew. They kept looking at me and I kept looking at them. Finally the lady came over to our table. "You were my husband's nurse. We were trying to figure out where we had seen you."

"Now I remember you," I said to her. Her husband looked over at me and smiled. I raised my voice a little so he could hear me and said, "I didn't recognize you with clothes on."

We really got some strange looks from the neighboring tables.

We all had a good laugh, but my face was red.

Happiness is . . . an easy day.

Things I wish could be changed:

Having a baby born with a little hook on the top of the head so the doctor can just slip his finger into it and gently pull the child out.

And after sixty having all people grow hooks on the side of their hips. Kind of like the ones on mattresses. Then if they break a hip, they will be so much easier to turn in bed.

Growing a third set of teeth after age fifty-five.

Identifying the flus with nicer names. Wouldn't you feel better with Paris Flu or Hawaiian Flu instead of Hong Kong or Asian Flu?

Happiness is . . . a smile and a "thank you" from a patient who has tried your patience all day.

One afternoon when I came on duty, I was told to go to the second floor. At report we heard that one of my ministers had his appendix out three days ago. He had not urinated since surgery, so the doctors still had to catheterize him.

"Okay, you go in and get your minister to 'piddle,' " I was told.

Thanks a lot. I went in and checked his temperature and blood pressure and asked him if he had used the bathroom.

"No," he replied. "I can't."

"How much have you had to drink today?" I asked.

"Not much," was his answer. "I hate to be catheterized, so I haven't drunk much. A few sips of water with my pills and a half cup of coffee." I left his room and returned shortly with a carafe of water and a bottle of 7-Up.

"Now you drink all this before tray time and you will be able to go." *Then I went out in the hall and said a little prayer.*

It was about 4:00 P.M. and trays come up at about 5:15. My thoughts were—fill up the bladder and it will be easier to go. *Also a strong positive thought: You will be able to go.* The doctors made rounds between five and six, so if he got really uncomfortable, they could catheterize him. In our hospital, nurses did not catheterize male patients. He emptied his bladder a little after five and was he thrilled. In his estimation I was a terrific nurse since I was the only one who helped him with his problem.

Happiness is . . . a very sick child gets well and goes home.

When I was dating my future husband, he and the minister discussed me. The minister was still raving about me. So, one of the first things my husband-to-be learned about me was that I was the best nurse to get you to "piddle." But he married me anyway!

Happiness is . . . never being spit up on, wet on, or bled on.

My "piddling" reputation keeps following me. One night when my new friend and I were eating out, we had a waitress who thought she knew me.

When she came to take our order, she said, "I think I know you, do you work in a doctor's office?"

"No," I replied, "I work at the hospital."

When she brought our salads, she said, "I wish I could remember where I met you."

She brought our main course with a big smile on her face. "I remember now. About two months ago, I had a baby. You were my nurse. You got me up to go to the bathroom, but you wouldn't leave me alone there. You said I might faint and you had to stay with me. I can't 'go' when someone else is in the bathroom. And still you wouldn't leave me. Well, I finally 'went' and you helped me back to bed."

It's very embarrasing to date when all the people I meet want to talk about 'piddling'.

Happiness is . . . a nursing mother and a hungry baby.

It really made me feel good when my nurse friends told my husband-to-be that he'd better be good to me or they would be after him.

But it really made my day when I met a patient whom I'd taken care of. She was coming to the hospital to have her third child in August. She was hoping I would be her nurse. I explained to her that I was getting married in April and would be retiring.

"Please come back because I didn't feel frightened

when you were there holding my hand and giving me encouragement."

Happiness is . . . "I'm glad you are my nurse to-night, I missed you last night."

Well, that's my story. Writing this book has brought back many memories—mostly good—of fellow nurses, doctors, and most importantly, the patients. I'm glad I became a nurse, but if I had my life to live over, I'm not sure I would have become a nurse. Maybe a librarian, that sounds like a slower pace—but I'd miss the babies.